THE ORIGINAL DEPRESSION HANDBOOK

A Complete Guide to Understanding
and Treating Depression

D1739197

Mark Liptak

I'M IN CRISIS!

Suicidal ideations require immediate attention.

If you or someone you know is in imminent danger:

* *

Dial: 911
Call the National Suicide Hotline

24/7 – Free – Confidential

1-800-SUICIDE (784-2433)

1-800-273-TALK (8255)

TTY/TDD Services

1-800-799-4 TTY (4889)

Use the Text Hotline

24/7 – Free – Confidential

In the To Line, Type: 741741

Use the Online Chat

Free - Confidential

IM-IN-Crisis.org

www.crisischat.org

TABLE OF CONTENTS

FOREWORD

The Original Depression Handbook: A Complete Guide to Understanding and Treating Depression was written for those who suffer every day quietly inside the confines of their own minds, either knowingly hiding their feelings or not even being aware that they are struggling with a major depressive disorder. In addition, *The Original Depression Handbook* is a reference guide to help depression sufferers gain control over their depression. It will also help family and friends have a better understanding of depression and how it affects those who suffer with it. Finally, *The Original Depression Handbook* illustrates the relationship between depression and suicide.

The incredible news about depression is that it can be controlled once properly diagnosed and treated. Once a treatment plan has been developed and implemented, you are on your way to regaining control of your mind and your life, and you will begin to live life like you never thought possible!

The Original Depression Handbook can be read from front to back, but it does not need to be. It is a reference book the chapters of which can be read in any order. You can choose which you wish to explore.

Due to the severity and overwhelming number of undiagnosed and untreated people who suffer from depression, it is my hope that *The Original Depression Handbook* will be part of everyone's homes, schools, libraries, medical institutions, doctors' offices, and counselors' offices.

You should know that depression goes by two other names: major depressive disorder and clinical depression. Whichever name is used, all three mean the same thing. **Depression = Major Depressive Disorder = Clinical Depression.**

Last, *The Original Depression Handbook* is a tool to help people have a better, clearer understanding of depression. If you are ready to begin a fuller, richer, more enjoyable life or to help someone who may be suffering from depression, let us get started.

CHAPTER I

An Overview of Depression

Depression has probably plagued mankind since man has been able to stand upright. Interestingly, prior to the nineteenth century people with depression were often thought to be possessed by demons. Today there is no doubt that depression is a leading affliction in our society and affects people in all walks of life regardless of age, sex, race, or socioeconomic status.

Who Can Benefit from *The Original Depression Handbook?*

The Original Depression Handbook was designed to provide individuals who suffer from depression, as well as their families and their friends, with a concise overview of depression. It is also intended to educate the reader on how depression can be tamed, if not conquered altogether. In addition, *The Original Depression Handbook* outlines how to develop a treatment plan for depression sufferers. If you are ready to begin a fuller, richer, more enjoyable life or to help someone suffering from depression, then let us get started.

Two Precepts to Agree to

A person with depression can employ many strategies that can help relieve the feelings of depression. While these feelings vary from person to person, they all have their roots in their ability to change the depressed person's thought process. Before we can discuss these strategies, you need to agree on two precepts.

1. **You must realize that you may be or are suffering from depression.**

2. **You must have a desire to feel better.**

If you agree to these two precepts, you are on your way to a better, more fulfilling life! If you do not agree with these two precepts, you may want to return this book before you damage too many more pages so you will be able to get a full refund. Got ya! Feel a little better already, don't you? See, you are already making progress!

If you do agree with these two precepts, then read on.

The Original Depression Handbook stresses how important it is for people who suffer with depression to be honest with themselves, their family, their friends, their physicians, and their counselors.

Please note a couple more things before you begin this journey. You need to know that there are no silver bullets for treating depression. As you will learn, depression treatments must be tailored to each individual. Also, remember that only a medical doctor can diagnose and treat depression.

Your doctor will help you find the right medications or combination of medications and can also guide you in finding the right

4

counselor. Finding the right medications and counselor may take some trial and error, but stick with it. You are worth it!

Facts about Depression

Most people may not be aware of numerous facts about depression. The following outlines some of these facts.

Depression affects all people regardless of age, race, gender, geographic location, demographic, or social position. (1)

Mental health disorders cost the global economy $1 trillion in lost productivity a year, with depression being the leading cause of ill health and disability, according to the World Health Organization. (1)

Depression is a common mental disorder. Globally, more than 264 million people of all ages suffer from depression. (2)

Approximately 80 percent of sufferers with depression are not receiving treatment. (3)

The total cost of depression in the United States is estimated to be $44 billion a year: $12 billion in direct costs for treatment, $8 billion in premature death, and $24 billion in absenteeism and reduced productivity at work. These numbers do not include out-of-pocket family expenses, costs of minor and untreated depression, excessive hospitalization, general medical services, and diagnostic tests. (4)

Depression is the leading cause of disability in the United States for people who are fifteen to forty-four years of age with 490 million disability days per year. (5)

Women are twice as likely to have depression and its symptoms compared to men of the same age. (5)

Participation in support groups when being treated for depression can increase treatment compliance by more than 85 percent. Support group participants are also more than 85 percent more willing to take their medication and cope with any side effects they may experience, which reduces inpatient hospitalizations. (5)

Data show about 25 percent of new prescriptions are never filled, and patients do not take their medications as prescribed about 50 percent of the time. (6)

Depression and anxiety disorders affect one in eight children in the United States. Children with this mental health issue are at a higher risk of performing poorly in school, having negative social experiences, and engaging in substance abuse. (5)

There are interrelationships between depression and physical health. For example, cardiovascular disease can lead to depression and vice versa. (2)

Up to 80 percent of people who are treated for depression will show improvement in their symptoms within four to six weeks of beginning a treatment plan. (5)

Eleven percent of children will have experienced the symptoms of a depressive disorder by the time they reach the age of eighteen. (5)

Thirty percent of college students report feeling depressed which disrupts their ability to function properly in school. (5)

Nearly 30 percent of people with substance abuse problems also suffer from depression. (7)

These facts about depression are startling when you consider how many people suffer with depression and may not even know why they feel the way they do.

CHAPTER 2

You Are Not Alone

You should know that if you do suffer from depression, you are not alone. A number of people from all walks of life had or have the same condition as you and still succeeded in life.

Let us take a quick look at a man we are all acquainted with—Abraham Lincoln. Lincoln suffered from depression but was still able to lead the United States through arguably the most difficult challenge it has ever faced.

Abraham Lincoln

According to Joshua Wolf Shenk, Lincoln's biographer,

> Lincoln experienced two major depressive breakdowns at age 26 and age 31, which included suicidal statements that frightened friends enough to form a suicide watch. When he was 32, Lincoln wrote, "I am now the most miserable man living." Lincoln's longtime law partner

William Herndon observed about Lincoln, "Gloom and sadness were his predominant state," and "His melancholy dripped from him as he walked." And another Lincoln friend reported, "Lincoln told me he felt like committing suicide often."

Even though Lincoln had depression, he was not totally crippled by it. In fact, it is possible that Lincoln's depression enabled him to see the world in a way only a person with a major depressive disorder could.

Depression Sufferers

The following is a list of people who suffer or have suffered with depression. While this is not an unabridged list, it is sufficiently long enough to help you realize that you are not alone and that depression affects many different people from many walks of life. Famous or not, these people are no different than you when it comes to living with depression.

Dwayne Johnson	Mark Twain	Winston Churchill
Kristen Bell	Nikola Tesla	Channing Tatum
Owen Wilson	Jim Carey	Richard Prior
Edgar Allan Poe	Billy Joel	Brad Pitt
Bill Murray	Andrew Lloyd Webber	Heath Ledger
Marie Osmond	Hans Christian Anderson	Mike Tyson
Howie Mandel	Alec Baldwin	Rosie O'Donnell
Frank Sinatra	Heather Locklear	David Letterman
Brooke Shields	John Lennon	Lady Gaga
Michael Jackson	Britney Spears	Alan Alda

Gwyneth Paltrow	Mark Liptak	Courtney Love
John Goodman	Marilyn Monroe	Johnny Cash
Johnny Carson	Virginia Wolf	Charles Darwin
Buzz Aldrin	Truman Capote	Terry Bradshaw
J. K. Rowling	Earnest Hemingway	Bob Dylan
Paul Getty	Mary Chapman Carpenter	Chevy Chase
Charles Dickens	Diana, Princess of Wales	Charles M. Schultz
Chris Farley	Marlon Brando	Beyoncé
Ray Charles	Emily Dickinson	Halle Berry
John Denver		

Depression did not start in the nineteenth century. Historical figures are also believed to have suffered with depression.

Vincent van Gogh	Michelangelo	Sir Isaac Newton
Ludwig von Beethoven	Julius Caesar	Napoleon Bonaparte
Wolfgang Amadeus Mozart		

Now that you realize that depression affects many people, it is also eye-opening to dispel the numerous myths concerning depression. Let us take a closer look at these myths.

CHAPTER 3

Depression Myths

Several myths or stigmas related to depression cause many of us to suffer in silence. Many people who do not understand depression believe these myths are true. The following are some of these myths.

Think Happy Thoughts. One myth is that depressed people only need to think themselves happy; if only that were true. We should "just snap out of it!" or "just get over it!"

Contagious. Some people fear depression might be contagious. The myth is if a person hangs around someone diagnosed with depression for too long, they might catch it. This simply is not true. It is more likely that the person already had or was at risk for depression. It is important to point out that while depression is not contagious, people can become burnt out from listening to a depressed person's complaints and may start avoiding them. Do not let your depression alienate you from people. Take action. You are worth it and so are they!

While depression is not "contagious," the act of suicide does appear to be "contagious." That is to say, there is a correlation between people who commit suicide and their family and friends becoming at higher risk of committing suicide themselves. More on this later.

Weak People. Another myth is that people with depression are weak people who should learn to be tougher and deal with life. This stigma can lead to dire consequences such as alcoholism, drug addiction, domestic violence, job loss, and even death.

Antidepressants Will Change My Personality. Antidepressant medications do not change one's personality—they simply do not work that way. They do help make you feel normal; that is to say, feel the same way as people who do not have depression feel.

Not a Real Disease. Perhaps the most limiting myth for treatment for depression is the myth that depression is not a real disease, like arthritis, cancer, or the flu. The myth is that depression is made up by doctors and pharmacological companies so they can make money treating us.

All You Need Is Prayer. This myth states that people with depression should be able to pray it away. Believers of this myth think of depression as a character flaw that can be fixed by following God's word. These well-meaning people do not understand that depression is a disease like cancer. Prayer is important; however, so are the God-gifted physicians who treat cancer. Simply telling people that they are depressed because of their current lifestyle or because of character flaws only exacerbates their depression.

It needs to be stated that God can heal, for those who believe, depression and any other disease He chooses. However, more often than not, He uses medical doctors to help us manage our depression.

As a disease, depression requires medical interventions including doctors, prescription medications, and counseling.

Finding out the truth about these myths will help you realize that your depression is a real disorder that needs to be treated. This leads us to our next topic: getting started on the path to understanding and treating depression.

CHAPTER 4

Defining Depression

The Mayo Clinic offers a simplified definition of depression: "Depression is a mood disorder that causes a persistent (greater than 2 weeks) feeling of sadness and loss of interest." Other names for depression are major depressive disorder and clinical depression.

The Three Names of Depression

Depression = Major Depressive Disorder = Clinically Depressed

Whichever name is used, depression can destroy your life if it goes untreated. It has led to divorce, job loss, family problems, and even death. Fortunately, depression can be treated with great success with doctor-prescribed medications, the support of family and friends, and counseling. As important as these strategies are for treating your depression, it has to start with you. We will get into the treatment of depression a little later on. For now, let us look at some of the different types of depression.

Types of Depression

Melancholic depression	Loss of pleasure in most or all activities
Atypical depression	Comfort eating weight gain, excessive sleep, significant social impairment
Catatonic depression	Rare and severe, unresponsive though awake, either immobile or exhibits bizarre movements
Anxious depression	Depression with sign and symptoms of anxiety
Postpartum depression	Experienced by 10 percent to 15 percent of women after childbirth
Seasonal affective disorder (SAD)	Comes in autumn or winter and resolves in spring
Bipolar depressive disorder	Depression is the low part, opposite the manic part, of bipolar disorder.
Persistent depressive disorder	Lasts for years; sufferers feel low and joyless most of the time, but can function day to day.
Situational depression	A major life event occurs such as the death of a loved one or the loss of a job.

Remember, only your doctor can diagnosis which specific type of depression you have. Some major depressive disorders last only a few months while others can last a lifetime. Let us take a look at some of these.

Temporary vs. Lifelong Depression

Note that some forms of depression, such as seasonal affective disorder and situational depression, are temporary. Seasonal affective disorder begins in the autumn or winter when people are exposed to diminished sunlight, causing a depletion in vitamin D. This depression resolves in the spring once exposure to the sun increases. The first line of defense for this type of depression is Vitamin D supplements.

Situational depression is another temporary form of depression. It comes on when a major life event occurs such as the loss of a job, divorce, or death of a loved one. This type of depression resolves when a new job is found or when the proper amount of time to mourn passes.

Others forms of depression, such as melancholic depression and persistent depressive disorder, can last a lifetime. Melancholic depression is where a person has lost all pleasure in most or all activities. Persistent depressive disorder can also last for years. The person feels low and joyless most of the time, but can still function day to day. Now that you have an idea of what depression is and what some of the different types of depression are, let us look at the feelings, signs, and symptoms associated with depression.

Are You Depressed?
Feelings Associated with Depression

One way to find out if you might be depressed is to write down how you have been feeling on a daily basis. Feelings common in people who have a depressive disorder are:

Tiredness	Irritability	Melancholy	Anger
Despair	Sadness	Loneliness	Paranoia
Suicidal ideations	Emptiness	Guilt	Stress
Hopelessness	Worthlessness	Insecurity	Frustration
Self-loathing	Unhappiness		

These feelings are not the exclusive property of depression. Almost everyone experiences many of these at some point in their lives. However, people who have a depressive disorder often experience many of these on a daily basis for greater than two weeks—even for years.

Signs and Symptoms of Depression

Another way to find out if you might be depressed is to write down any signs and symptoms you may be experiencing on a daily basis. Signs and symptoms often associated with depression are:

Self-harm	Lack of energy	No motivation
Loss of interest	Difficulty concentrating	Sleeping too much
Chronic exhaustion	Isolating yourself	Sleeping too little
Chronic headaches	Eating habit changes	Argumentative
Chronic body pains	Diminished concentration	Suicide attempts
Frequent yelling	Pretending to be happy	Short-tempered
Poor grades	Missing school	Being bullied
Frequent crying	Continual unhappiness	Believing you are better off dead

Again, these signs and symptoms are not the exclusive property of depression. Most people experience many of these sometimes. People with a depressive disorder suffer any number of these on a daily basis for longer than two weeks when depression is gone untreated.

On the next two pages are charts you can use to track your feelings, signs, and symptoms of depression that you may experience over the next fourteen days.

Feelings Associated with Depression Chart														
	1	2	3	4	5	6	7	8	9	10	11	12	13	14
Anger														
Crying														
Despair														
Emptiness														
Frustration														
Guilt														
Hopelessness														
Insecurity														
Irritability														
Loneliness														
Melancholy														
Paranoia														
Sadness														
Self-loathing														
Stress														
Tiredness														
Unhappiness														
Worthlessness														

Signs and Symptoms Associated with Depression Chart														
	1	2	3	4	5	6	7	8	9	10	11	12	13	14
Argumentative														
Believing you are better off dead														
Chronic body pains														
Chronic exhaustion														
Chronic headaches														
Continual unhappiness														
Diminished concentration														
Eating habit changes														
Frequent yelling														
Isolating yourself														
Lack of energy														
Loss of interest														
No motivation														
Self-harm														
Short-tempered														
Sleep too little														
Sleep too much														
Suicide ideations														
Suicide attempts														
Frequent crying														
Pretending to be happy														

Testing for Depression

Another, more scientific method to discover if you might be depressed is to take a simple test. Everyone should take a test like this. Go on. You might learn something about yourself.

A number of quick, free depression tests are available on the Internet for you to try. The following page has one taken from the following website:

https://www.healthyplace.com/depression/
depression-information/depression-test-free-online-depression-test

Depression Screening Test

For this free online depression screening test, think about your mood and activities over the past two weeks. Note whether you agree or disagree with the following depression test questions.

1. I have felt a low or depressed mood almost every day.

2. I have lost all interest in activities I used to find pleasurable.

3. My weight or appetite has significantly changed.

4. My sleep has been disturbed.

5. I find myself feeling restless or slowed down.

6. I have no energy.

7. I feel worthless.

8. I find focusing or making decisions difficult.

9. I keep thinking about death or suicide.

10. I feel rejected by others.

11. These feelings cause significant distress and negatively impact my day-to-day life.

Depression Test Scoring

If you answered "agree" to five or more of these depression test statements, including statements 1, 2, or both, you may be depressed. Note that depression is only typically diagnosed when it negatively impacts day-to-day functioning—in other words, answering "agree" to statement 11.

If this free online depression test suggests you are depressed, you should see a professional healthcare provider for a medical assessment for a mood disorder. Please note that this online depression test is not designed to rule out other diseases and only a medical doctor can diagnose depression.

Remember that taking a test is only a preliminary indicator of whether you have a major depressive disorder. Only a medical doctor can diagnose and treat depression.

Now that we have defined depression, looked at the feelings, signs, and symptoms related to depression, and have taken a depression test, you should have a good idea of what depression is, what it looks like, and if you are at risk for depression. Next let us see what causes depression.

CHAPTER 5

What Causes Depression?

Many doctors believe that depression occurs due to a chemical imbalance in our brains. The chemicals believed to affect our moods are the neurotransmitters serotonin, norepinephrine, and dopamine. For years doctors have been prescribing antidepressant medications that help increase these neurotransmitters' levels in the brain in order to treat depression.

Chemical imbalances in the brain, however, vary from individual to individual. This is why finding the right medication or combination of medications can be challenging. The following is a brief list of what can cause chemical imbalances in the brain.

Causes of Depression

Chronic Pain	Lack of sunlight	Stressful life events
Medications	Poor nutrition	Physical health problems

| Hormonal changes | Grief and loss | Faulty mood regulation |
| Postpartum | Substance abuse | Genetics |

As previously stated, limited amounts of the neurotransmitters serotonin, norepinephrine, and dopamine appear to play a major role in depression. To correct for these limited amounts of neurotransmitters, several types of medications have been developed that are thought to increase the amount of these neurotransmitters in the brain. These medications do not simply add neurotransmitters to the brain. They work by stopping the brain from reabsorbing neurotransmitters, thus creating more available neurotransmitters. These medications are known as selective reuptake inhibitors (SRIs). Let us look at how this all works.

The Ship Analogy

Think of neurotransmitters as ships that move around in the liquid part of your brain. Their job is to stabilize the good feelings we have by keeping the brain chemically balanced. These ships occasionally stop at docking ports, known as synapses of the brain, which send messages to the brain. The synapses are like marinas attached to nerve cells known as neurons. Some of the ships docked at the marina are reabsorbed into the neurons. In normal brain activity, this is not a problem. New ships replace the ones that have been reabsorbed.

People with depression also have these ships. Unfortunately, the number of new ships does not offset the number of ships that are reabsorbed. Therefore, there are fewer ships to appropriately maintain the good, stable feelings in the brain, and the person can develop feelings of depression.

While the lack of ships can create or exacerbate the feelings that lead to depression, medications can be prescribed that slow down the rate of reabsorption. These SRI medications inhibit the reabsorption of the ships, thus maintaining a strong fleet of ships, aka neurotransmitters.

Antidepressants

In some cases only one antidepressant medication is enough to treat the symptoms of depression. In others it may take two, three, or more of these medications used simultaneously. As there are so many different antidepressants and varying levels of depression, finding the right medication regimen might take some time. So do not get discouraged if the first antidepressant you are prescribed does not fully treat the symptoms of your depression.

The following is a list of common antidepressants. You can see that different SRIs work differently on the three neurotransmitters: serotonin, norepinephrine, and dopamine. This is why finding the right antidepressant medication regimen can be challenging.

Names and Types of Common Antidepressants

Trade Name	Clinical Name	Type of Antidepressant
Celexa	Citalopram	Selective serotonin reuptake inhibitor (SSRI)
Lexapro	Escitalopram	SSRI
Prozac	Fluoxetine	SSRI
Luvox	Fluvoxamine	SSRI
Paxil	Paroxetine	SSRI
Zoloft	Sertraline	SSRI
Seroquel	Quetiapine	SSRI
Zyprexa	Olanzapine	SSRI

Rexulti	Brexpiprazole	SSRI
Trintellix	Vortioxetine	SSRI
Cymbalta	Duloxetine	Serotonin and norepinephrine reuptake inhibitor (SNRI)
Effexor	Venlafaxine	SNRI
Pristiq	Desvenlafaxine	SNRI
Khedezla	Esvenlafaxine	SNRI
Fetzima	Levomilnacinran	SNRI
Wellbutrin	Bupropion	Norepinephrine and dopamine reuptake inhibitor (NDRI)
Abilify	Aripiprazole	Antipsychotic (increases serotonin and dopamine)
Desyrel	Trazadone	Monoamine oxidase inhibitor (MAOI) (increases norepinephrine, serotonin, and dopamine)
Remeron	Mirtazapine	Tetracyclic (faster-acting; increases serotonin, norepinephrine, and dopamine)

While medication may be the first line of defense for treating depression, you can do several other things to help with your depression. More on this later. First let us examine what happens when we self-medicate or stop taking our prescribed antidepressant medications all at once.

CHAPTER 6

Self-Medicating

Considering that up to 80 percent of people suffering from depression are not being treated, a reasonable question is, how many of the untreated suffers of depression are not even aware they are self-medicating with nicotine, alcohol, and drugs? Taking this question a step further, how many alcoholics or people addicted to recreational drugs are actually suffering from depression and if their depression was properly treated could stop smoking, drinking to excess, or taking nonprescription drugs?

You may notice when you start taking antidepressant medications that you are smoking less, drinking less, or have stopped using nonprescription drugs to treat your depression. You will simply feel better and no longer need to self medicate.

Antidepressant medications will work only as long as you keep taking them regularly. Do not stop taking them without specific instructions from your primary care provider, and you should never stop taking them abruptly.

Stopping Your Antidepressant Medications

Once you have been on an antidepressant medication regimen for several months or even for years, you may decide to stop taking them. You may be feeling so mentally stable that you do not believe you need them anymore. This is not only foolish, but could even be dangerous. Discontinuing your antidepressant medication regimen without consulting your physician is never a good idea. If you do want to stop taking them, you need to know that these medications need to be tapered off to avoid possible side effects, and you must always notify your primary care physician prior to stopping them.

Withdrawal Syndrome

The name for stopping your antidepressant medication abruptly is *discontinuation syndrome*. Some doctors use the more appropriate term *withdrawal syndrome*. Withdrawal syndrome is more appropriate in that it connotes the seriousness of stopping your medications abruptly.

The View defines withdrawal as "the group of physical and mental symptoms that occur when a person abruptly stops or decreases their intake of medications or recreational drugs. The symptoms usually only occur after a person has developed dependence on a drug or drugs". (8)

Signs and symptoms of withdrawal syndrome differ drastically from person to person. The severity of the withdrawal syndrome is usually worse the longer you have been on antidepressant medications.

Rebound Depression

One problem that can occur is called rebound depression. This is when the signs and symptoms of your depression come back, for several weeks, worse than before you started your antidepressant medication regimen due to the abrupt changes in your brain's chemical makeup.

Brain Zaps

Another problem that can occur is called brain zaps. Sometimes brain zaps are referred to as brain shivers, brain shocks, or head shocks. They are described as one of the most unbearable withdrawal symptoms when stopping certain antidepressant and antianxiety medications. Brain zaps get their name from the uncomfortable sensations they cause, which are described as sudden zaps, electrical buzzes, tremors, shakes, or jolts in the brain. (9)

The following is a list of common signs and symptoms of withdrawal syndrome.

Withdrawal Symptoms

Panic attacks	Rebound depression	Tremors
Fever	Brain zaps	Anxiety
Confusion	Ataxia (lack of muscle control)	Nausea
Hallucinations	Lightheadedness	Diarrhea
Headaches	Anger	Dizziness

Not only is stopping your antidepressant medication regimen dangerous, but you could lose all the ground you have made. You will start having all the same feelings, signs, and symptoms of being depressed. These feelings may not return all at once; this will probably occur over time while the effects of the antidepressants gradually leave your body.

Antidepressant Medications Take Effect

Antidepressants can take four to six weeks to take their full effect on your brain, and they can take weeks to clear out of your system. In the end, you will be miserable and may find yourself self-medicating with alcohol, recreational drugs, or cigarettes again. If you are fortunate, you may have someone in your life who will reopen your eyes to your daily misery and encourage you to get back on your medications.

Stopping your antidepressant medications is just as bad as stopping any prescribed medications. For instance, you would never stop taking your high blood pressure medication without first contacting your doctor. Keep in mind: if we did not need our prescription medications, our doctors would not have prescribed them to us.

Do not be like the 50 percent of people who will become noncompliant with their antidepressant medication regimen. Stay on the medications your doctor has prescribed you. They are an essential part of your treatment plan.

As good as medication is for treating depression, it is only one part of a successful treatment plan for depression. The next chapter brings all the pieces of a complete treatment plan together.

CHAPTER 7

Plan of Treatment

The very first thing you must do in developing a plan of treatment is to be honest with yourself. Nothing can happen without you!

Getting started will probably be the hardest part of the process. Unless you are willing to be honest about your feelings and the signs and symptoms you are experiencing, your doctor will not be able to diagnose that you are depressed or what type of depression you are suffering with. Do not let social myths and stigmas keep you hiding your depression from your doctor as you probably have tried to do with your family and friends. Being open and honest is the first step in recovery.

Your Role

As stated earlier, you must begin by being 100 percent honest with yourself. Write down your feelings, signs, and symptoms as they occur. Include the time of day in your notes as this will help your doctor discern any patterns and help get you started on the best anti-depressant medication regimen to treat your specific symptoms.

Doctor's Role

Here again, you need to be 100 percent honest with your primary care physician or your psychiatrist. Otherwise, you will be wasting your time as well as the time of your doctor. Don't be ashamed. Your doctor will understand. The importance of a medical doctor cannot be overstressed. Your doctor will take the information you have provided about your depression and decide what medication or combination of medications will work best to treat your depression. In addition, your doctor will help you navigate treatment options for depression that you may not even know about.

For instance, there is a relatively new procedure called genetic testing. Genetic testing uses your DNA to help your doctor find the best medication regimen to treat your specific depression. While this technique is not needed for everyone, it is an example of a tool at the disposal of your doctor that you may have had no idea that it was an option.

Medication

Doctor-prescribed antidepressants are often the first part of a treatment plan. While there may be some trial and error in establishing an antidepressant medication regimen, antidepressants are an integral part of your overall treatment plan. Remember, no two brains are exactly alike. No two antidepressant plans of treatment will be exactly alike either.

Counselor's Role

Finding a counselor who specializes in mood disorders and who is right for you may take some time. You will need to find a counselor you feel comfortable with and can trust. Counselors do not only listen to you. They will give you individualized tools to help you manage your ongoing bouts of depression.

Counselor is a broad term that encompasses psychiatrists, psychologists, and social workers. While both psychologists and social workers are excellent counselors, psychiatrists are medical doctors who can prescribe medications in addition to providing counseling.

Family and Friends

Although some depression sufferers do not have the support of family or friends, organizations such as those mentioned in the "I'm in Crisis!" section found in the front of this handbook can fill this void.

If you are a family member or a friend of a person who is depressed, you can take several steps to help them get the treatment they need. First and foremost, love them unconditionally. While this can be challenging at times, it is so important.

Other steps you can take include being patient and understanding with what they are going through. Remember they are suffering from a disease they are struggling to deal with. Be willing to discuss their problem with them. Be honest with them and tell them what you are seeing them do and hearing them say.

If you suspect they are in crisis, reach out to the National Suicide Hotline, Text Hotline, or online chat for guidance. If the situation calls for it, be willing to call 911. This is discussed in greater detail in Chapter 8.

Diversions from Depression

Now that you are being honest with yourself, have a doctor, are on an antidepressant medication regimen, found a counselor, and have the support of your family and friends, your depression is now 100 percent cured, right? Unfortunately, no. You are still going to have some bad days. For depression comes and goes in waves. Like waves, times of depression have different heights of disability and the length of stays are uncertain.

Fortunately, these days will not be as dim or all consuming as they were before you began seeking help. Also, you can do things on those days to help you feel less depressed. These suggestions are intended to divert your mind from depressive thoughts by filling it with positive thoughts so the negative thoughts cannot fit in. These diversions will help you avoid the slippery slope of depression. The following list gives examples of things you can do when you are feeling depressed.

Exercise	Play with your pet	Go shopping
Read a book	Talk with a friend	Pray
Place reaffirming sticky notes around your home	Join an online discussion group	Say positive things about yourself to yourself
Avoid negative conversations, news, and people	Socialize. Get out of your home. Visit family or friends.	Practice good hygiene and dress nicely
Meditate	Listen to music	Take up a hobby
Watch a funny video	Watch a movie	Have consensual sex
Take a nap	Sing	Dance
Read the Bible	Play a musical instrument	Write a book
Draw cartoons	Color pictures	Join a church
Go bowling	Join a league	Paint a picture
Go for a drive	Go out to dinner	Ride your motorcycle
Write in a journal	Go fishing	

Let us look at all the pieces of a successful depression treatment plan in the form of a simple formula.

Recipe for Treating Depression

Honest with yourself + Doctor + Medication + Counseling + Family and friends + Diversions = Controlled depression

While the recipe for treating depression appears easy to follow, in reality it will take a major commitment from you to establish your treatment plan. You will still need to work at keeping your depression in check.

CHAPTER 8

Depression and Suicide

It would be remiss if *The Original Depression Handbook* did not address the relationship between depression and suicide. In fact, according to JasonFoundation.com, 60 percent of all people who commit suicide suffer from depression, and that figure jumps to 90 percent for teenagers. In addition to depression, other risk factors associated with suicide include the following:

Other mental illnesses	Alcohol abuse	Drug abuse
Bullying	Puberty	LGBTQ community
Self-mutilation	Violence in the home	Family history of suicide
Unwanted pregnancy	Native American /Alaskan youth	Low self-esteem
Learning disabled	Previous attempts	Sexually transmitted disease
Financial loss	Rejection by peers	Sexual abuse
Job loss	Death of loved one	Divorce
Loss of relationship	Perfectionist personality	Chronic pain

Signs and Symptoms of Suicidal Ideations

As you can see, there is no one reason why people commit suicide. In addition to the risk factors associated with suicide, other signs can be seen in almost 90 percent of people who commit suicide. Let us take a look at these.

Most people who are having suicidal ideations—that is to say thoughts of suicide—often discuss it out loud by stating things such as: "I am going to kill myself." "What's the use? I'm worthless anyway." "I just can't deal with it anymore." "I'm fine. I have it all worked out. I know exactly what I need to do." Although it may seem odd that a person will be this open with their suicidal ideations, many people contemplating suicide openly state these types of things.

Another sign that a person may be contemplating suicide is they may suddenly become calm and relaxed after years, months, or weeks of being depressed. This could be a sign that they have made the decision to end their life as the answer to their continual suffering.

Other signs that a person may be considering suicide include the following. They start giving away their most cherished possessions. They call all their family and friends and tell them goodbye. They display increased irritability or aggression. They withdraw from family and friends. They start taking excessive risks or they may be preoccupied with death. Any of these is a sign that some sort of intervention could be needed.

Suicidal Ideation Myths

As with depression, several myths around suicidal ideation need to be dispelled.

Talking about Suicide. One myth is that people who talk about suicide will not really do it. The fact is, many people considering suicide actually do discuss it. It may be in a normal conversation or, as stated previously, they may make statements such as "I would be better off dead."

Suicidal Ideation. Another myth is if you ask someone if they are having suicidal ideations that you are putting this idea into their heads. This is also not true and actually a good question to ask to help prevent suicides or suicide attempts. People who are contemplating suicide are often looking for another answer. Asking them if they are having suicidal ideations opens a window of opportunity to discuss their feelings and reasons why they are considering suicide.

No Way to Stop Suicides. Yet another myth is that there is no way to stop someone once they have decided to commit suicide. Suicides and attempted suicides can be stopped in many cases with intervention such as medications that treat their depression, counseling, family support, and diversionary tactics similar to those used to treat depression. Sometimes just having someone to talk to can make the difference between life and death.

Even though there are ways to prevent someone from committing suicide, sometimes people cannot be saved. They simply do not have the reasoning power or the support groups needed to stop themselves. This is the reason why family, friends, and support groups are so important and why everyone needs to become acquainted with the signs of depression that can lead to suicide when gone untreated.

Facts about Suicide

According to the University of Texas, 75 percent of people who commit suicide are depressed. (10)

Close to eight hundred thousand people die of suicide every year. Suicide is the second leading cause of death in fifteen to twenty-nine year-olds with accidents being the first. (2)

Almost 80 percent of all suicides are male. (11)

Females attempt suicide more than three times as often as males; however, males die by suicide more than four times as often as the females. (12)

Ten teenagers out of one hundred thousand decide to kill themselves. (13)

A silent epidemic is sweeping through our nation that claims an average of more than one hundred twenty-five young lives each week. (14)

In the ten-to-twenty-four age group, 81 percent of suicide deaths were males and 19 percent were females. (14)

Cultural variations also exist in suicide rates. Native American/ Alaskan Native youth have the highest rates of suicide-related fatalities. (14)

Caucasian youth have the second highest rate of suicide. (14)

African-American youth have the third highest rate of suicides. (14)

Alcohol and drug use, which clouds judgment, lowers inhibitions, and worsens depression, is associated with 50–67 percent of suicides. (14)

More teenagers and young adults die from suicide than from cancer, heart disease, AIDS, birth defects, stroke, pneumonia, influenza, and chronic lung disease combined. (14)

Each day in the United States of America alone, there is an average of more than 3,069 attempts of suicide by young people in grades nine through twelve. (14)

Four out of five teens who attempt suicide have given clear warning signs. (14)

One death by suicide occurs every twelve minutes in the United States alone. (15)

Research shows that approximately 90 percent of people who have dies by suicide were suffering from a mental illness at the time. The most common mental illness reported was depression. (16)

Untreated depression is the number one risk for suicide among youth, especially teen boys. The ratio of suicide is seven to one for teen boys with untreated depression compared to teen girls. (15)

Approximately two hundred and fifty thousand people become suicide survivors each year. (17)

Suicide Prevention

Given that 75 percent of people who commit suicide are depressed, it is important to recognize the symptoms of depression so they can be treated appropriately.

In addition, the warning signs of suicide need to be taken seriously. If you see or hear any of the warning signs, ask the person if they are thinking about committing suicide. This will not push them to follow through with their suicidal ideation. It will actually help to prevent them from following through with it and open a dialog with them about their current feelings.

Another option for people contemplating suicide or for people trying to help someone is to contact a suicide help line and ask them for direction. You can do this by calling, texting, or opening a chat session with a number of help groups such as the ones listed in the "I'm in Crisis!" section found in the front of this handbook. In any event, you need to do something.

Remember approximately 80 percent of people who suffer with depression are not receiving treatment. This obviously leaves a huge number of people who may be depressed and by extension be at risk of committing suicide. By bringing up your awareness of the signs and symptoms of depression you can better understand depression and offer help to individuals who are contemplating suicide. You just may save a life.

CHAPTER 9

Summation

Hopefully, *The Original Depression Handbook* has helped you, your family members, and your friends have a clearer understanding of depression and has shown you the steps required to treat it effectively.

You

If you suffer from depression and have gotten one useful bit of information out of this handbook, please share it with your family and friends. *The Original Depression Handbook* will help them have a better understanding of what you are going through.

Family and Friends

If you purchased *The Original Depression Handbook* to have a better understanding of what someone with depression is going through and found it a useful tool for learning about depression, then please share it with a person you suspect may by suffering from depression or who has already been diagnosed with depression.

With all the medical knowledge and alternatives to treat depression, there is no longer any reason that depression cannot be effectively managed except when it goes undiagnosed. By following the steps outlined in *The Original Depression Handbook* you will discover if you may be suffering from depression, and if you are, have a means to establishing a treatment plan. Remember, the first step to a happier, more fulfilling life starts with you!

BIBLIOGRAPHY

(1) Adam Jezard, "Depression Is the No. 1 Cause of Ill Health and Disability Worldwide", World Economic Forum, May 18, 2018, https://www.weforum.org/agenda/2018/05/depression-prevents-many-of-us-from-leading-healthy-and-productive-lives-being-the-no-1-cause-of-ill-health-and-disability-worldwide

(2) "Depression", World Health Organization, January 30, 2020, https://www.who.int/news-room/fact-sheets/detail/depression

(3) Emma Carlson Berne, "Depression", Farmington Hills, MI: The Gale Group, 2007, https://www.factretriever.com/depression-facts

(4) Raymond W. Lam, and Hiram Wok. "Depression", New York, NY: Oxford University Press, 2008, https://www.factretriever.com/depression-facts

(5) Louise Gaille, "44 Surprising Depression Statistics", Vittana Personal Finance Blog.org, March 16, 2017, https://vittana.org/44-surprising-depression-statistics

(6) Jane Brody, "The Cost of Not Taking Your Medicine", The New York Times, April 17, 2017, https://www.nytimes.com/2017/04/17/well/the-cost-of-not-taking-your-medicine.html

(7) Virginia Edwards, M.D., "Depression and Bipolar Disorders: Everything You Need to Know", Buffalo, NY:Firefly Books Inc., 2002

(8) "Drug Withdrawal Definition", The View, 2019, https://theviewsc.com/drug-withdrawal-definition/

(9) Jillian Levy, "Brain Zaps Plus 4 Brain Zaps Natural Remedies", October 31, 2018, https://draxe.com/health/brain-zaps/

(10) "Teen Suicide Overview", Teen Suicide Statistic, 2021, http://teensuicidestatistics.com/

(11) Mark Baird, "White Male Suicide Epidemic In America", Hirepatriots, January 23, 2019, https://hirepatriots.com/white-older-men-suicides

(12) Nancy Schimelpfening, "Differences In Suicides Among Men and Women", Verywell Mind, November 16, 2020, https://www.verywellmind.com/gender-differences-in-suicide-methods-1067508

(13) Brian Resnick, "A Promising New Clue to Prevent Teen Suicide: Empower Adults Who Care", Vox, February 28, 2019, https://www.vox.com/science-and-health/2019/2/28/18234667/teen-suicide-prevention

(14) "Higher Risk Groups", The Parent Resource Program, The Jason Foundation, 2021, http://prp.jasonfoundation.com/facts/youth-suicide-statistics/

(15) "Depression Facts", Hope for Depression Research Foundation, 2021, https://www.hopefordepression.org/depression-facts/

(16) "Suicide In Teens and Children Signs and Causes", Boston Children's Hospital, 2021, https://wwwchildrenshospital.org/conditions-and treatments/conditions/s/suicide-and-teens/symptoms-and-causes

(17) "Suicide Survivors Share Their Letters to the Departed", The Columbus Dispatch, November 21, 2015, https://www.dispatch.com/article/20151120/NEWS/311209653